UNRAVELING MULTIPLE SCLEROSIS

A Comprehensive Guide to Diagnosis, Treatment, and Living Well

Dr. Raymond F. Bernard

TABLE OF CONTENTS

CHAPTER 1

Multiple Sclerosis

Imagine a complex system of electrical wires, each responsible for transmitting important messages throughout your home. These wires need to be insulated and protected to ensure a smooth flow of information. Similarly, in our bodies, we have a sophisticated communication network known as the nervous system. It's like the wiring of our body, consisting of billions of nerve cells called neurons. This nervous system, particularly the central nervous system (CNS), is essential for our ability to move, think, and perceive the world around us.

Multiple sclerosis (MS) is a medical condition that disrupts this intricate communication network. It's a chronic autoimmune disease that affects the CNS, causing a wide range of physical and cognitive symptoms. In this chapter, we will dive into the world of multiple sclerosis, its historical context, its prevalence, and why early diagnosis and treatment are crucial.

Understanding the Basics of Multiple Sclerosis

At its core, multiple sclerosis is a disease that targets the central nervous system. The CNS comprises the brain and spinal cord, and it plays a central role in controlling various bodily functions. Think of the CNS as the control center for your entire body, responsible for sending and receiving messages that regulate everything from walking and talking to sensing pain and processing emotions.

In a healthy CNS, nerve cells, or neurons, communicate effectively through a fatty substance called myelin. Myelin acts like insulation around the nerve fibers, allowing electrical impulses to travel quickly and smoothly along the neurons. This ensures that when your brain signals your hand to move, for example, the message arrives promptly and the movement occurs without hitches.

However, in multiple sclerosis, something goes wrong with this vital communication system. The immune system, which normally protects the body from harmful invaders like bacteria and viruses, mistakenly attacks the myelin sheath. This attack causes inflammation, damages the myelin, and disrupts the transmission of electrical signals along the nerves. As a result, the messages between the brain and other parts of the body become disrupted or even blocked entirely.

A Historical Perspective on Multiple Sclerosis

The history of multiple sclerosis dates back centuries. The first recorded description of MS-like symptoms can be traced to the ancient Greeks and Romans. However, it wasn't until the 19th century that significant progress was made in understanding the condition.

In 1868, French neurologist Jean-Martin Charcot made groundbreaking contributions to the field of neurology by extensively studying and categorizing MS. He helped distinguish MS from other neurological diseases and identified the characteristic patterns of the disease. Charcot's work laid the foundation for future research and paved the way for a better understanding of MS.

Throughout the 20th century, scientific advancements,

particularly in medical imaging and immunology, deepened our understanding of MS. The development of techniques like magnetic resonance imaging (MRI) allowed for the visualization of CNS lesions, aiding in the diagnosis and monitoring of the disease.

The Global Impact of Multiple Sclerosis

Multiple sclerosis is not limited to a specific geographical region or population. It affects people around the world, although its prevalence can vary based on factors such as genetics and environmental influences.

Globally, it is estimated that over 2.8 million people live with MS. The prevalence is notably higher in regions further from the equator, suggesting a possible link between MS and vitamin D levels, which are influenced by sunlight exposure. In countries with temperate climates, the prevalence of MS is generally higher than in tropical regions.

Despite these geographical differences, MS is a global health concern, and its impact extends beyond individual patients.

Families, friends, and communities are all affected, as they provide support and care for those living with the condition.

The Importance of Early Diagnosis and Treatment

In the world of medicine, timing is often critical, and multiple sclerosis is no exception. Early diagnosis and timely intervention can make a significant difference in the course of the disease and the quality of life for individuals living with MS.

The early stages of multiple sclerosis often involve relapses, or episodes of worsening symptoms, followed by periods of remission, during which symptoms improve or even disappear. Identifying and diagnosing MS during these early stages is crucial because effective treatments are available to manage the disease and reduce the frequency and severity of relapses.

Diagnostic tools such as MRI scans, cerebrospinal fluid analysis, and clinical evaluations by neurologists play a pivotal role in the early detection of MS. These tools help confirm the presence of the disease, rule out other conditions with similar symptoms, and provide valuable insights into the extent of CNS damage.

Once diagnosed, individuals with MS can work with healthcare providers to develop a personalized treatment plan. This plan may include disease-modifying therapies (DMTs) that can slow the progression of the disease and reduce the frequency of relapses. Physical therapy, occupational therapy, and lifestyle modifications are also important components of MS management, aimed at maintaining mobility and overall well-being.

In summary, multiple sclerosis is a complex neurological condition that disrupts the central nervous system's ability to function properly. It has a rich history of scientific exploration and understanding, dating back to the ancient world but significantly advancing in the 19th and 20th centuries. MS has a global impact, affecting millions of individuals and their communities, and its prevalence can vary based on geographical and environmental factors. Early diagnosis and intervention are crucial for managing the disease effectively and improving the quality of life for those living with MS. As we continue our journey through the chapters of this book, we will explore the various aspects of multiple sclerosis in more depth, from its different forms and causes to its symptoms and management strategies.

CHAPTER 2

Understanding the Nervous System

The nervous system is one of the most intricate and vital systems in our bodies. It's the master conductor that orchestrates every move we make, thought we have, and sensation we feel. To truly grasp multiple sclerosis (MS) and its impact, we must first understand the nervous system and its inner workings. In this chapter, we will delve into the anatomy and function of the central nervous system (CNS), the role of the immune system in CNS protection, and how MS disrupts this delicate balance.

The Central Nervous System: Our Body's Command Center

Picture the central nervous system (CNS) as the epicenter of a bustling city, with countless roads and pathways connecting all its parts. The CNS consists of two key components: the brain and the spinal cord. The brain, encased within the skull, is our body's command center. It's responsible for processing information from our senses, making decisions, and coordinating all our bodily functions.

The spinal cord, which runs from the base of the brain down the back, serves as the CNS's main highway. It acts as a relay between the brain and the rest of the body, transmitting signals to control everything from muscle movement to heart rate. The spinal cord is protected by the bony vertebral column, making it less vulnerable to external injury.

The Role of Neurons: Messengers of the Nervous System

At the heart of the nervous system are neurons, specialized cells that transmit electrical and chemical signals. Neurons are like messengers, delivering important information throughout the body. They come in various shapes and sizes but share a common structure: a cell body, dendrites, and an axon.

- **Cell Body:** The cell body contains the nucleus and other vital components that keep the neuron alive and functioning.
- **Dendrites:** These branch-like extensions receive

signals from other neurons or sensory receptors and transmit them to the cell body.

- **Axon:** The long, slender axon carries signals away from the cell body to other neurons, muscles, or glands.

To ensure efficient communication, neurons are coated with a fatty substance called myelin. Myelin acts like insulation around electrical wires, allowing nerve impulses to travel rapidly and smoothly along the axon. Think of myelin as the protective coating on an electrical cord, ensuring that the signals reach their destination intact and without interference.

The Immune System's Role in CNS Protection

The central nervous system is a delicate and vital structure, and the body has evolved multiple mechanisms to protect it. One such mechanism is the blood-brain barrier (BBB), a specialized barrier that separates the circulating blood from the brain and spinal cord tissue. The BBB is like a strict customs checkpoint, allowing only certain substances to pass into the CNS while keeping harmful agents out.

The immune system also plays a role in CNS protection. While the immune system's primary job is to defend the body against infections and foreign invaders, it must carefully regulate its activities within the CNS to avoid causing harm. The CNS has its own immune system known as microglia, which are specialized immune cells that patrol the brain and spinal cord, removing damaged cells and responding to threats.

How MS Disrupts the Nervous System

Now, let's discuss how MS, an autoimmune disease, disrupts this intricate system. As previously mentioned, MS occurs when the immune system mistakenly attacks the myelin sheath that coats neurons within the CNS. This misguided attack triggers inflammation, damaging the myelin and disrupting the normal flow of electrical impulses.

The immune system's attack on myelin in MS leads to the formation of lesions or plaques within the CNS. These are areas of damaged or scarred myelin and may also involve damage to the underlying nerve fibers. Imagine these lesions as potholes on a road, causing disruptions and slowing down the transmission of signals along the nerve fibers.

The location and extent of these lesions can vary widely among individuals with MS, which explains the diverse range of symptoms associated with the disease. Depending on where the lesions develop, individuals may experience issues with mobility, coordination, sensation, cognition, or other bodily functions.

It's important to note that MS is a chronic disease characterized by periods of relapse and remission. During a relapse, new symptoms may appear or existing ones may worsen due to the inflammation and demyelination processes. Remission, on the other hand, is a period of partial or complete recovery, often facilitated by the body's ability to repair some of the damaged myelin.

However, over time, repeated relapses and remissions can lead to accumulated damage within the CNS, resulting in progressive disability. This is why early diagnosis and intervention are so critical in managing MS; they aim to slow down the disease's progression and minimize disability.

In summary, the nervous system, particularly the central nervous system (CNS), is the body's communication network, with neurons as its messengers. Neurons transmit signals along axons, coated with myelin, which ensures efficient communication. The immune system, including the blood-brain barrier and microglia, plays a crucial role in protecting the CNS. Multiple sclerosis disrupts this system by causing the immune system to attack the myelin sheath, leading to inflammation, lesions, and disrupted nerve function. Understanding the basics of the nervous system and how MS affects it is essential for comprehending the complexities of this disease, which we will explore further in the subsequent chapters of this book.

CHAPTER 3

Types of Multiple Sclerosis

Multiple sclerosis (MS) is a complex and diverse disease that manifests in various forms. Understanding the different types of MS is essential for both patients and healthcare providers as it helps guide treatment decisions and prognostic discussions. In this chapter, we will explore the primary types of MS, each with its own characteristics and disease course, as well as some rare variants and subtypes.

1. Relapsing-Remitting MS (RRMS)

Relapsing-remitting MS (RRMS) is the most common form of the disease, accounting for approximately 85% of all cases. It is characterized by distinct episodes of neurological symptoms called relapses or exacerbations, followed by periods of partial or complete recovery known as remissions.

During a relapse, new symptoms may emerge, or existing ones may worsen, typically lasting for days to weeks. These episodes are often unpredictable and can be triggered by various factors, including stress or infections. The recovery phase, or remission, can last for varying durations, and some individuals may return to their baseline level of function, while others may experience residual symptoms.

Over time, many individuals with RRMS transition to a secondary-progressive form of the disease, known as secondary-progressive MS (SPMS), in which there is a gradual accumulation of disability with or without continued relapses.

2. Secondary-Progressive MS (SPMS)

Secondary-progressive MS (SPMS) typically follows the initial relapsing-remitting phase. In SPMS, there is a steady accumulation of disability over time, with or without the occurrence of relapses. This transition can be gradual, and not everyone with RRMS will progress to SPMS.

SPMS can manifest in various ways. Some individuals may

experience occasional relapses with sustained disability progression, while others may have a more gradual and continuous worsening of symptoms. The unpredictability and variability of SPMS make it challenging to manage, emphasizing the importance of early intervention with disease-modifying therapies (DMTs) during the RRMS phase to potentially delay or mitigate the progression to SPMS.

3. Primary-Progressive MS (PPMS)

Primary-progressive MS (PPMS) is less common than RRMS but is often considered more disabling from the onset. Unlike RRMS, PPMS is characterized by a steady and gradual worsening of symptoms without distinct relapses or remissions. The progression in PPMS may be more linear, making it difficult to identify specific exacerbation periods.

Diagnosing PPMS can be challenging, as its progression can resemble other neurological conditions. It typically manifests in adulthood and is more prevalent among slightly older individuals compared to RRMS. Managing PPMS is particularly challenging because there are limited approved treatments available specifically for this subtype. Symptomatic management, rehabilitation, and support are essential components of care for people with PPMS.

4. Progressive-Relapsing MS (PRMS)

Progressive-relapsing MS (PRMS) is one of the rarer forms of the disease, accounting for a small percentage of cases. This subtype is characterized by a steady progression of disability from the onset, similar to PPMS, but with superimposed relapses or exacerbations.

Unlike RRMS, where relapses are typically followed by periods of remission, individuals with PRMS experience a continuous progression of symptoms with relapses that do not lead to significant recovery. PRMS is often challenging to manage due to its aggressive and relentless nature, and it may require a multifaceted approach that combines symptom management, rehabilitation, and experimental treatments.

Rare Variants and Subtypes

In addition to the primary types of MS mentioned above, there are several rare variants and subtypes that present unique challenges and considerations:

1. Pediatric MS: While MS is more commonly diagnosed in adults, it can also affect children and adolescents. Pediatric MS has its own set of challenges, including differential diagnosis, treatment considerations, and addressing the educational and emotional needs of young patients.

2. Radiologically Isolated Syndrome (RIS): RIS refers to the incidental finding of abnormalities on brain imaging, such as MRI, in individuals who do not yet have clinical symptoms of MS. It poses a diagnostic dilemma, as not all individuals with RIS will go on to develop MS. Close monitoring and clinical evaluation are necessary to determine if and when treatment is needed.

3. Benign MS: Some individuals with MS experience minimal disability progression over many years, despite having the disease. This form of MS is often referred to as benign MS. While it may seem less severe, it still requires careful monitoring, as progression can occur later in life.

4.   Fulminant   MS: This extremely rare and aggressive form of MS progresses rapidly and severely, leading to significant disability within a short period. Management of fulminant MS is challenging, and treatment approaches may involve high-dose immunosuppression.

Conclusion: The Complexity of MS Subtypes

Multiple sclerosis is not a one-size-fits-all condition. Its various subtypes and manifestations highlight the complex nature of the disease. Each individual's journey with MS is unique, and the course of the disease can be highly variable.

Diagnosing and categorizing MS subtypes is essential for tailoring treatment plans and interventions to the specific needs and challenges of each patient. Early diagnosis and appropriate treatment, especially during the relapsing-remitting phase, can significantly impact the course of the disease and help individuals with MS lead fulfilling lives.

As we continue our exploration of multiple sclerosis in this book, we will delve deeper into the causes and risk factors that contribute to the development of MS, further understanding its symptoms and the diagnostic process, and exploring the management strategies and advancements in research and treatment that offer hope to individuals living with this complex condition.

CHAPTER 4

Causes and Risk Factors

Multiple sclerosis (MS) is a complex and multifactorial disease, and while its exact cause remains elusive, researchers have made significant progress in understanding the factors that contribute to its development. In this chapter, we will explore the current knowledge regarding the potential causes and risk factors associated with MS, shedding light on the interplay between genetics, environmental influences, and immune system dysfunction.

Genetic Factors: The Role of Genetics in MS

Genetics plays a significant role in the susceptibility to multiple sclerosis. While MS is not directly inherited in a Mendelian fashion (i.e., it doesn't follow a simple dominant or recessive inheritance pattern), having a family member with MS does increase an individual's risk of developing the disease.

Several genetic variants have been identified that are associated with an increased risk of MS. The most notable genetic risk factor is the HLA-DRB1 gene, part of the human leukocyte antigen (HLA) complex, which plays a crucial role in immune system regulation. Variations in the HLA-DRB1 gene are thought to contribute to an individual's susceptibility to autoimmune diseases, including MS.

However, having these genetic risk factors does not guarantee that someone will develop MS. Many individuals with these genetic markers never develop the disease, highlighting the importance of other factors in MS development.

Environmental Factors: Triggers and Associations

While genetics set the stage, environmental factors appear to trigger or influence the onset of MS in genetically susceptible individuals. These environmental factors can vary widely and may include:

1. Vitamin D: There is a strong association between vitamin D deficiency and an increased risk of MS. Vitamin D plays a crucial role in immune system regulation, and low levels have been linked to a higher susceptibility to autoimmune diseases. Some studies suggest that exposure to sunlight, which enables the body to produce vitamin D, may be protective against MS. However, the relationship between vitamin D and MS is complex and not fully understood.

2. Infections: Certain viral and bacterial infections have been investigated for their potential role in MS development. Epstein-Barr virus (EBV), for example, is more common in individuals with MS than in the general population. It is believed that infections like EBV may trigger an abnormal immune response in genetically susceptible individuals, leading to the development of MS.

3. Smoking: Smoking is a well-established environmental risk factor for MS. Smokers have a higher risk of developing the disease compared to non-smokers. The exact mechanisms by which smoking contributes to MS risk are still under investigation, but it is believed to involve the harmful effects of smoking on the immune system and inflammation.

4. Geography and Climate: MS is more prevalent in regions farther from the equator, which receive less sunlight and have lower average vitamin D levels. This geographical distribution suggests a potential role of environmental factors related to latitude and climate in MS risk.

Immune System Dysfunction: The Key Player

At the core of MS is an abnormal immune response. In individuals with MS, the immune system mistakenly identifies myelin, the protective covering of nerve fibers, as a foreign invader and launches an attack against it. This immune system dysfunction is the hallmark of autoimmune diseases, and in the case of MS, it results in inflammation, demyelination, and damage to the central nervous system.

The precise triggers for this immune system malfunction in MS remain a subject of ongoing research. It's likely that a combination of genetic susceptibility and environmental exposures creates a perfect storm, leading to an aberrant immune response against the body's own tissues.

The Complexity of MS Etiology

It's important to recognize that multiple sclerosis is a multifaceted disease with no single cause. Instead, it's influenced by a complex interplay of genetic, environmental, and immune system factors. This complexity explains why MS affects individuals differently, with a wide range of symptoms and disease courses.

Moreover, MS is considered a polygenic disease, meaning that multiple genes are involved in its development. The interaction of these genes with environmental factors further complicates the picture. Researchers have identified over 200 genetic risk variants associated with MS, highlighting the genetic complexity of the disease.

The Role of Epstein-Barr Virus (EBV)

Among the various environmental factors linked to MS, the Epstein-Barr virus (EBV) has garnered significant attention. EBV is a common herpesvirus that causes infectious mononucleosis, also known as glandular fever. It's estimated that over 90% of people worldwide are infected with EBV at some point in their lives.

Several lines of evidence suggest a strong association between EBV and MS:

1. **Higher Prevalence in MS Patients:** Studies have consistently shown a higher prevalence of EBV infection in individuals with MS compared to the general population.

2. **Timing of Infection:** Many individuals with MS have evidence of EBV infection before the onset of MS symptoms. This suggests

that EBV infection may be a trigger for the development of MS in genetically susceptible individuals.

3. **EBV-Specific Immune Response:** Abnormalities in the immune response to EBV have been observed in individuals with MS, suggesting that the virus may play a role in driving the autoimmune response seen in the disease.

While these findings are intriguing, the exact mechanisms by which EBV contributes to MS development are still being investigated. It's important to note that EBV is just one of many factors believed to be involved in MS, and more research is needed to fully understand its role.

Conclusion: The Complex Interplay of Causes and Risk Factors

Multiple sclerosis is a complex and multifactorial disease with a range of genetic, environmental, and immune system factors contributing to its development. Genetics set the stage, environmental factors act as triggers or influencers, and immune system dysfunction is at the core of the disease.

Understanding the interplay between these factors is crucial for advancing our knowledge of MS and developing more effective treatments and prevention strategies. While there is no single cause of MS, ongoing research continues to uncover the intricate mechanisms that drive this complex condition.

As we progress through this book, we will delve further into the diagnosis of MS, exploring the common symptoms and the diagnostic process that enables healthcare providers to identify the disease. Additionally, we will explore the various strategies and therapies available for managing MS and improving the quality of life for individuals living with this condition.

CHAPTER 5

Symptoms and Diagnosis

Multiple sclerosis (MS) is a highly variable condition, and its symptoms can range from mild to severe, affecting different parts of the body and mind. In this chapter, we will explore the common symptoms of MS and the diagnostic process, which plays a crucial role in identifying the disease and guiding treatment decisions.

Common Symptoms of Multiple Sclerosis

The symptoms of MS can be diverse and unpredictable, as they depend on the location and extent of damage within the central nervous system (CNS). Some of the most common symptoms of MS include:

1. Fatigue: Fatigue is one of the most prevalent and debilitating symptoms of MS. It can range from mild to severe and often interferes with daily activities. MS-related fatigue is not solely due to physical exhaustion but is also linked to the disease's impact on the brain and nervous system.

2. Muscle Weakness: Weakness in the limbs, particularly in the legs, is a common symptom of MS. This can lead to difficulty with walking and other physical activities. Weakness may be intermittent, occurring during relapses, or it can progressively worsen in the case of progressive forms of MS.

3. Numbness and Tingling: Many individuals with MS experience numbness, tingling, or a pins-and-needles sensation in various parts of the body. These sensations are often temporary and can affect the face, arms, legs, or trunk.

4. Balance and Coordination Problems: MS can disrupt the brain's ability to coordinate movements and maintain balance, leading to problems with walking and a higher risk of falls.

5. Vision Changes: Visual disturbances are common in MS and can include blurred vision, double vision (diplopia), eye pain, and even temporary vision loss. Optic neuritis, inflammation of the optic nerve, is a frequent manifestation.

6. Cognitive Changes: MS can affect cognitive functions such as memory, attention, and problem-solving. Some individuals may experience difficulties with multitasking and processing information.

7. Spasticity: Muscle stiffness and spasms are common in MS, often leading to discomfort and pain. Spasticity can affect mobility and interfere with daily activities.

8. Bowel and Bladder Dysfunction: MS can disrupt the normal functioning of the bowel and bladder, leading to issues such as constipation, urinary urgency, and incontinence.

9. Pain: Chronic pain, including headaches and musculoskeletal pain, is prevalent in individuals with MS. Pain can result from muscle spasms, nerve damage, or other MS-related factors.

10. Emotional and Mood Changes: Depression, anxiety, and mood swings are common in MS. Coping with a chronic condition, as well as the physical and cognitive challenges it presents, can contribute to emotional distress.

It's important to note that not every person with MS will experience all these symptoms, and the severity and combination of symptoms can vary widely. Additionally, some individuals may experience symptom exacerbations (relapses) followed by periods of partial or complete symptom improvement (remissions), while others may have a more progressive course of disease with gradual worsening of symptoms.

The Diagnostic Process

Diagnosing multiple sclerosis can be challenging, as its symptoms can mimic those of other neurological conditions. The diagnostic process typically involves a combination of clinical evaluation, imaging studies, and laboratory tests. Here's a breakdown of the steps involved:

1. Medical History and Clinical Examination: A neurologist will review the patient's medical history and conduct a thorough neurological examination. The neurologist will assess sensory and motor function, coordination, reflexes, and cranial nerve function.

2. Magnetic Resonance Imaging (MRI): MRI is a crucial tool in diagnosing MS. It can reveal the presence of lesions or plaques in the central nervous system, which are characteristic of the disease. These lesions appear as areas of abnormal signal intensity on MRI scans.

3. Cerebrospinal Fluid Analysis: In some cases, a lumbar puncture (spinal tap) may be performed to analyze cerebrospinal fluid (CSF). Elevated levels of certain proteins and the presence of specific immune cells in the CSF can provide supportive evidence of MS.

4. Evoked Potentials: Evoked potential tests measure the electrical activity in the brain in response to sensory stimuli, such as visual or auditory stimuli. Abnormalities in these tests can indicate CNS dysfunction.

5. Clinical Criteria: The McDonald criteria are a set of diagnostic criteria used to establish a diagnosis of MS. These criteria take into account clinical symptoms, imaging findings, and the presence of CSF abnormalities.

6. Exclusion of Other Conditions: To confirm a diagnosis of MS, other conditions that can mimic MS must be ruled out. These include neuromyelitis optica (NMO), acute disseminated encephalomyelitis (ADEM), and other demyelinating disorders.

Early Diagnosis and the Importance of Treatment

Early diagnosis of MS is crucial for several reasons:

1. Treatment Initiation: Starting treatment early in the course of the disease can help manage symptoms, reduce the frequency and severity of relapses, and potentially slow down the progression of disability. Disease-modifying therapies (DMTs) are often prescribed to individuals with MS, and their effectiveness is maximized when initiated early.

2. Symptom Management: Early diagnosis allows for prompt symptom management, addressing issues such as fatigue, pain, and spasticity to improve the individual's quality of life.

3. Emotional Support: An early diagnosis provides individuals with MS and their families the opportunity to access support and resources for coping with the emotional and psychological challenges that can accompany the condition.

4. Lifestyle Modifications: Early diagnosis enables individuals to make necessary lifestyle modifications, such as incorporating regular exercise, a healthy diet, and stress management techniques into their daily routines.

In summary, multiple sclerosis is characterized by a wide range of symptoms that can affect various aspects of a person's life. Diagnosis is based on a combination of clinical evaluation, imaging studies like MRI, laboratory tests, and adherence to diagnostic criteria. Early diagnosis is essential for initiating treatment and support, ultimately improving the long-term outcomes for individuals living with MS. As we continue our journey through this book, we will explore various aspects of MS, including its different forms and causes, as well as strategies for managing the condition and emerging research and treatment options.

CHAPTER 6

Managing Multiple Sclerosis

Multiple sclerosis (MS) is a lifelong condition that requires comprehensive management to address its diverse and often unpredictable symptoms. In this chapter, we will explore various aspects of managing MS, including medications for symptom management and disease modification, lifestyle and dietary considerations, and the role of physical therapy and rehabilitation.

Medications for Symptom Management

While there is no cure for MS, several medications and therapies are available to manage its symptoms and improve the quality of life for individuals with the condition. Symptom management is a critical aspect of MS care, as it helps alleviate the discomfort and challenges associated with the disease. Here are some common symptoms and the medications used to manage them:

1. Relapse Treatment: During relapses or exacerbations, when new symptoms or a worsening of existing symptoms occur, corticosteroids such as methylprednisolone are often prescribed. These drugs can help reduce inflammation and speed up recovery.

2.   Disease-Modifying Therapies (DMTs): DMTs are a group of medications that aim to modify the course of the disease by reducing the frequency and severity of relapses. They are used primarily in relapsing forms of MS. Examples of DMTs include interferon beta, glatiramer acetate, and newer oral and infusion therapies.

3. Muscle Spasticity: Medications such as baclofen, tizanidine, and dantrolene may be prescribed to alleviate muscle stiffness and spasms.

4. Pain Management: Depending on the type and severity of pain, various medications, including nonsteroidal anti-inflammatory drugs (NSAIDs), anticonvulsants, and opioids, may be used to manage pain in MS.

5. Fatigue: Medications such as amantadine or modafinil may be prescribed to address fatigue in MS. However, non-pharmacological strategies like energy conservation techniques and lifestyle modifications are also important for managing fatigue.

6. Bladder and Bowel Dysfunction: Medications and strategies to manage bladder issues include anticholinergic medications for overactive bladder and intermittent catheterization for urinary retention. Bowel dysfunction may be addressed with dietary changes, medications, and bowel training.

7. Depression and Anxiety: Psychotherapy, counseling, and medications such as selective serotonin reuptake inhibitors (SSRIs) and serotonin-norepinephrine reuptake inhibitors (SNRIs) are used to manage mood disorders commonly associated with MS.

8. Cognitive Symptoms: Cognitive rehabilitation, including strategies to improve memory, attention, and problem-solving, is often recommended to address cognitive deficits.

9.   Painful   Symptoms:
Neuropathic pain in MS may be managed with medications like gabapentin or pregabalin.

It's important for individuals with MS to work closely with their healthcare providers to develop a personalized treatment plan that addresses their specific symptoms and needs. Medications should be monitored for effectiveness and potential side effects, and adjustments may be made as necessary.

Lifestyle and Dietary Considerations

Managing MS extends beyond medications; lifestyle and dietary choices also play a significant role in overall well-being. Here are some key considerations:

1. Diet: A balanced and nutritious diet is essential for maintaining overall health. While there is no specific MS diet, some individuals find that dietary modifications, such as reducing saturated fats and increasing intake of omega-3 fatty acids, can help manage inflammation. Others may benefit from specific diets, such as the Mediterranean diet, which is rich in fruits, vegetables, and healthy fats.

2. Exercise: Regular physical activity can help improve strength, flexibility, and balance, which can be especially beneficial for individuals with MS. It can also help combat fatigue and boost mood. Physical therapists can provide guidance on exercise routines tailored to individual abilities and needs.

3. Stress Management: Stress can exacerbate MS symptoms and contribute to relapses. Stress-reduction techniques such as meditation, mindfulness, yoga, and relaxation exercises can help manage stress and improve overall well-being.

4.   Smoking   Cessation: Smoking is a known risk factor for MS and can worsen the disease's progression. Quitting smoking is an important step in managing the condition.

5. Sun Exposure and Vitamin D: Vitamin D deficiency has been linked to an increased risk of MS and disease progression. Adequate sun exposure, dietary sources of vitamin D, and supplements, when recommended by a healthcare provider, can help maintain optimal vitamin D levels.

6. Sleep: Quality sleep is essential for overall health and well-being. Individuals with MS should address sleep disturbances and aim for a regular sleep schedule.

Physical Therapy and Rehabilitation

Physical therapy and rehabilitation are integral components of managing MS, as they focus on maintaining and improving mobility, function, and independence. Here's how they can benefit individuals with MS:

1. Mobility and Gait Training:
Physical therapists work with individuals to improve balance and coordination, enhance strength and flexibility, and address gait abnormalities. Assistive devices such as canes, walkers, and braces may be recommended.

2. Occupational Therapy:
Occupational therapists help individuals with MS learn strategies to perform daily activities more independently. They can recommend assistive devices and techniques to

overcome challenges in tasks such as dressing, cooking, and bathing.

3. Speech and Swallowing Therapy: For individuals with MS experiencing speech or swallowing difficulties, speech therapists can provide exercises and techniques to improve communication and prevent aspiration.

4. Cognitive Rehabilitation: Cognitive rehabilitation programs help address cognitive deficits by providing strategies to improve memory, attention, and problem-solving skills.

5. Fatigue Management: Occupational therapists can teach energy conservation techniques and pacing strategies to manage fatigue effectively.

6. Aquatic Therapy: Aquatic therapy in a heated pool can help individuals with MS improve strength, flexibility, and balance while reducing the impact on joints and muscles.

7. Assistive Technology: Rehabilitation specialists can assess individuals' needs for assistive devices and technology, such as mobility aids, adaptive computer equipment, and home modifications, to enhance independence.

Emotional and Psychological Support

Living with MS can take an emotional toll, and addressing the psychological aspects of the condition is essential for overall well-being. Mental health professionals, such as psychologists or counselors, can provide support and therapy to help individuals cope with the emotional challenges of MS, including depression, anxiety, and adjustment to the diagnosis.

Support Groups and Resources

Joining MS support groups or connecting with advocacy organizations can provide individuals and their families with valuable resources, information, and a sense of community. Support groups offer opportunities to share experiences, exchange advice, and receive emotional support from others facing similar challenges.

In conclusion, managing multiple sclerosis is a multifaceted process that involves medication, lifestyle and dietary considerations, physical therapy, rehabilitation, and emotional support. It's essential for individuals with MS to work collaboratively with their healthcare providers to develop a comprehensive treatment plan tailored to their specific needs and symptoms. With the right management strategies and support, individuals with MS can lead fulfilling lives and effectively navigate the challenges of this chronic condition. As we continue our exploration of MS in this book, we will delve into emerging research and treatment options, as well as strategies for living well with MS.

CHAPTER 7

Emerging Research and Treatment Advances in Multiple Sclerosis

Multiple sclerosis (MS) is a dynamic field of research and medical advancement. In this chapter, we'll explore the exciting developments and treatment advances that offer hope to individuals living with MS. From cutting-edge therapies to promising research directions, this chapter delves into the future of MS care.

1. Disease-Modifying Therapies (DMTs): The Evolving Landscape

Over the years, the landscape of disease-modifying therapies (DMTs) for MS has evolved significantly. DMTs are at the forefront of MS treatment, and researchers are continuously working to improve their effectiveness, safety, and accessibility. Some notable trends and advancements include:

A. Oral and Infusion Therapies: Newer oral and infusion therapies have expanded treatment options, providing alternatives to traditional injectable DMTs. These options offer convenience and potentially improved adherence for individuals with MS.

B. Personalized Medicine: Researchers are exploring the concept of personalized medicine in MS treatment. This approach tailors therapy to an individual's specific disease characteristics, genetic factors, and treatment responses. The goal is to optimize treatment outcomes while minimizing side effects.

C. Therapies for Progressive Forms: Historically, treatment options for progressive forms of MS have been limited. However, there are now DMTs specifically approved for primary-progressive MS (PPMS) and secondary-progressive MS (SPMS). Ongoing research is focused on identifying effective treatments for these forms of the disease.

D. Repair and Remyelination Therapies: Beyond managing inflammation and relapses, researchers are exploring therapies that promote repair and remyelination in the central nervous system (CNS). These treatments aim to restore damaged myelin and improve function.

2. Emerging Therapies and Clinical Trials

The MS research community is actively investigating novel therapeutic approaches to address the complex nature of the disease. Promising areas of research and emerging therapies include:

A. Stem Cell Therapies: Stem cell transplantation is being explored as a potential treatment for MS. Researchers are investigating various types of stem cells and transplantation techniques to promote CNS repair and modulate the immune system.

B.   Neuroprotection: Neuroprotection strategies aim to safeguard nerve cells and prevent further damage in MS. These approaches involve medications and interventions that target mechanisms of cell injury and death.

C. Gut Microbiome: Emerging research suggests a connection between the gut microbiome and MS. Investigating the role of gut bacteria in immune regulation and inflammation may lead to novel treatment approaches, such as probiotics or dietary interventions.

D. Repurposed Drugs: Some existing medications that were originally developed for other conditions are being repurposed for MS treatment. This approach can expedite the availability of potential therapies.

E. Advanced Imaging Techniques: Advances in imaging technology, such as advanced MRI techniques, are enabling researchers to better visualize and understand the disease's progression. These imaging tools are vital for monitoring treatment responses and assessing disease activity.

3. Precision Medicine and Biomarkers

Precision medicine, which tailors treatment to an individual's unique characteristics, is gaining traction in MS research. Biomarkers, specific biological indicators, are being studied to predict disease progression, treatment response, and relapse risk. These markers can guide treatment decisions, allowing for more personalized and effective care.

4. Telemedicine and Remote Monitoring

The COVID-19 pandemic accelerated the adoption of telemedicine in MS care. Telehealth allows individuals with MS to access healthcare remotely, reducing barriers to regular check-ups and consultations. Remote monitoring tools, including wearable devices and smartphone apps, enable individuals to track their symptoms and share data with healthcare providers for better disease management.

5. Wellness and Lifestyle Interventions

Complementary approaches to MS management are gaining recognition. Lifestyle interventions, including diet, exercise, stress reduction, and mindfulness, are being studied for their impact on symptom management and overall well-being. Integrating these strategies into MS care can enhance quality of life.

6. Collaborative Research Efforts

International collaboration among researchers, healthcare providers, advocacy organizations, and individuals with MS is fostering a robust research environment. Large-scale research initiatives, data sharing, and patient registries are accelerating the pace of discovery and facilitating the development of more effective treatments.

7. Patient-Centered Care

Patient-centered care is becoming increasingly central to MS management. Individuals with MS are encouraged to actively participate in their treatment decisions, share their goals and preferences, and collaborate with healthcare providers to develop personalized care plans.

8. Access to Treatment and Healthcare Equity

Ensuring equitable access to MS treatments and care is a critical focus in the field. Efforts are being made to address disparities in access, especially among underserved populations, and to advocate for policies that promote affordability and accessibility of treatments.

9. Future Directions in Research

The future of MS research holds promise in several key areas:

A.   Precision   Medicine: Advancements in understanding the genetic and immune system factors underlying MS will drive the development of more personalized treatments.

B. Combination Therapies: Researchers are exploring the potential benefits of combining different DMTs or treatment modalities to maximize efficacy while minimizing side effects.

C. Long-Term Outcomes: Long-term studies are essential to assess the safety and effectiveness of treatments over extended periods, particularly in progressive forms of MS.

D. Neurorepair: Strategies to promote neural repair and remyelination remain a major focus, with the goal of restoring lost function.

E. Preventive Strategies: Research into preventive measures, such as vaccines or early interventions, is ongoing to reduce the risk of developing MS.

Conclusion: A Brighter Future for MS

The landscape of multiple sclerosis research and treatment is rapidly evolving. Emerging therapies, precision medicine, remote monitoring, and patient-centered care are shaping the future of MS management. With the dedication of researchers, healthcare providers, and advocacy organizations, individuals with MS can look forward to improved treatments, enhanced quality of life, and the hope of a cure on the horizon. As we continue our exploration of MS in this book, we will delve deeper into the lived experiences of individuals with MS, provide guidance on navigating the challenges of the condition, and offer insights into building resilience and maintaining a positive outlook in the face of adversity.

CHAPTER 8

Living Well with Multiple Sclerosis

Living with multiple sclerosis (MS) can be challenging, but it is possible to lead a fulfilling and meaningful life. In this chapter, we will explore strategies and insights to help individuals with MS navigate the physical, emotional, and practical aspects of their daily lives, promoting well-being and resilience.

1. Self-Care and Symptom Management

Managing MS starts with self-care and symptom management. Here are some essential self-care strategies:

A. Medication Adherence: Taking prescribed medications consistently is vital for controlling symptoms and slowing disease progression. Setting up reminders and working closely with healthcare providers can facilitate adherence.

B. Healthy Lifestyle: Eating a balanced diet, engaging in regular exercise, staying hydrated, and getting adequate sleep are fundamental to overall health. These lifestyle factors can also help manage some MS symptoms, such as fatigue and muscle stiffness.

C. Stress Management: Chronic stress can exacerbate MS symptoms. Stress-reduction techniques, including meditation, yoga, mindfulness, and deep breathing exercises, can help individuals manage stress effectively.

D. Fatigue Management: Managing fatigue is a key aspect of self-care in MS. Pacing activities, taking breaks, and prioritizing rest can help conserve energy and reduce fatigue.

E. Temperature Sensitivity: Many individuals with MS are sensitive to temperature changes. Avoiding extreme heat and using cooling strategies, such as cooling vests and staying hydrated, can help manage heat sensitivity.

2. Building a Support Network

A strong support network is invaluable for individuals with MS. This network may include:

A. Healthcare Team: Developing a collaborative relationship with healthcare providers, including neurologists, physical therapists, and mental health professionals, is essential. Open communication can help address concerns and adapt treatment plans as needed.

B. Family and Friends: Loved ones can provide emotional support, assist with daily tasks, and accompany individuals to medical appointments. Educating family and friends about MS can foster understanding and empathy.

C. Support Groups: Joining MS support groups or online communities can connect individuals with others facing similar challenges. Sharing experiences, advice, and coping strategies can reduce feelings of isolation.

D. Advocacy Organizations: MS advocacy organizations provide resources, information, and advocacy opportunities. They also play a crucial role in raising awareness and advancing research.

3. Navigating Everyday Challenges

Living with MS involves addressing various daily challenges:

A. Mobility and Accessibility: Adapting the home environment for mobility aids, such as ramps or grab bars, can enhance safety and independence. Additionally, individuals with MS may need to explore accessible transportation options.

B. Employment: Managing work-related challenges, including fatigue, cognitive symptoms, and physical limitations, may require accommodations or adjustments to work schedules. Open communication with employers is key.

C. Financial Planning: MS can incur significant medical expenses. Financial planning, including health insurance considerations and budgeting, is essential to ensure access to necessary care and support.

D. Maintaining Independence: Assistive devices, such as mobility aids or adaptive technology, can help individuals with MS maintain independence in daily activities.

4. Emotional Well-Being

The emotional impact of MS can be profound. Here are some strategies for promoting emotional well-being:

A. Seeking Counseling: Professional counseling or therapy can help individuals cope with the emotional challenges of MS, including depression, anxiety, and grief.

B. Expressing Emotions: Sharing feelings with loved ones or through creative outlets like journaling, art, or music can provide a healthy emotional release.

C. Mindfulness and Meditation: Practicing mindfulness and meditation techniques can help individuals stay grounded and reduce emotional distress.

D. Setting Realistic Goals: Setting achievable goals, both short-term and long-term, can provide a sense of purpose and accomplishment.

5. Nurturing Relationships

Maintaining healthy relationships is crucial for emotional well-being:

A. Communication: Open and honest communication with loved ones about MS-related challenges and needs is essential for nurturing relationships.

B. Intimacy: MS may impact sexual function and intimacy. Communicating with partners and exploring adaptive strategies can help maintain intimacy.

C. Social Engagement: Staying socially engaged with friends and family, even when physical limitations are present, can combat feelings of isolation.

6. Future Planning and Resilience

Planning for the future is essential for individuals with MS:

A. Advance Directives: Creating advance directives, including healthcare proxies and living wills, ensures that healthcare decisions align with personal preferences.

B. Financial Planning: Long-term financial planning, including retirement and estate planning, can provide peace of mind for the future.

C. Building Resilience: Resilience involves adapting to challenges and setbacks.

Developing resilience through positive coping strategies can help individuals thrive despite the uncertainties of MS.

7. Staying Informed and Advocating for MS

Being well-informed about MS and advocating for oneself is empowering:

A. MS Education: Continuously learning about MS, including treatment options, research advances, and self-care strategies, helps individuals make informed decisions.

B. Advocacy: Becoming an advocate for MS research, awareness, and policy changes can contribute to positive change in the MS community.

C. Clinical Trials: Staying informed about clinical trials and research opportunities allows individuals to explore potential new treatments and contribute to the advancement of MS knowledge.

Conclusion: Thriving with Multiple Sclerosis

Living well with MS involves a holistic approach that addresses physical, emotional, and practical aspects of life. By prioritizing self-care, building a strong support network, and developing resilience, individuals with MS can thrive and lead fulfilling lives despite the challenges of the condition. As we conclude our exploration of MS in this book, we hope to leave you with a sense of hope and empowerment in the face of MS, emphasizing that a fulfilling and meaningful life is not only possible but achievable for those living with this condition.

CHAPTER 9

Understanding and Supporting Loved Ones with Multiple Sclerosis

Multiple sclerosis (MS) doesn't just affect the individual diagnosed; it also has a significant impact on their loved ones—spouses, partners, family members, and friends. In this chapter, we will explore the challenges faced by caregivers and provide insights into understanding, supporting, and caring for someone with MS while also taking care of oneself.

1. Understanding Multiple Sclerosis

To effectively support someone with MS, it's crucial to have a basic understanding of the condition. MS is an unpredictable autoimmune disease that affects the central nervous system, leading to a wide range of symptoms and varying degrees of disability. It can impact mobility, cognition, energy levels, and emotional well-being. However, MS is highly variable, and no two individuals experience it in the same way.

Understanding the unpredictable nature of MS is the first step in providing empathetic support. The disease can be characterized by periods of remission and exacerbation, meaning symptoms may come and go. Some individuals may experience mild symptoms, while others may face more severe challenges.

2. The Role of Caregivers

Caregivers play a critical role in the lives of individuals with MS. They provide emotional support, assist with daily tasks, accompany their loved ones to medical appointments, and often become advocates for their care. Caregiving can be both rewarding and demanding, and it's important for caregivers to recognize the significance of their role.

3. Challenges Faced by Caregivers

Caring for someone with MS can be emotionally and physically taxing. Here are some common challenges faced by caregivers:

A. Emotional Impact: Witnessing a loved one's struggles with MS can evoke a range of emotions, including sadness, frustration, anxiety, and grief. It's essential for caregivers to acknowledge and address their emotional well-being.

B. Balancing Roles: Caregivers often juggle multiple roles, including that of a partner, parent, employee, and caregiver. Finding a balance between these roles can be challenging.

C. Physical Demands: Assisting with mobility, personal care, and household tasks can be physically demanding. Caregivers may experience fatigue and strain.

D. Communication: Effective communication is vital, but it can be challenging when both the caregiver and the individual with MS are dealing with the emotional impact of the disease.

E. Self-Care: Caregivers may neglect their own self-care as they prioritize the needs of their loved ones. This can lead to burnout and decreased well-being.

4. Providing Support and Empathy

Supporting a loved one with MS requires empathy, patience, and open communication. Here are some ways to provide effective support:

A. Active Listening: Take the time to listen to your loved one's thoughts, concerns, and feelings. Allow them to express themselves without judgment.

B. Learn Together: Explore resources, attend educational sessions, or accompany your loved one to medical appointments. Understanding the condition can help both of you make informed decisions.

C. Encourage Independence: While it's essential to offer assistance, encourage your loved one to maintain as much independence as possible. Let them take the lead when they can.

D. Be Flexible: MS symptoms can fluctuate, and daily routines may need to adapt. Flexibility is key in accommodating changing needs.

E. Share Responsibilities: If possible, involve other family members or friends in caregiving responsibilities. Sharing the load can prevent caregiver burnout.

5. Self-Care for Caregivers

Taking care of oneself is not selfish; it's essential for providing effective care to a loved one with

MS. Here are some self-care strategies for caregivers:

A. Seek Support: Reach out to support groups, counseling services, or therapist to help manage your own emotional well-being.

B. Maintain Your Health: Prioritize your physical health by eating well, getting regular exercise, and ensuring you have adequate rest.

C. Set Boundaries: Establish clear boundaries to balance your caregiving role with your personal life and responsibilities.

D. Respite Care: Arrange for respite care or breaks to recharge and prevent caregiver burnout.

E. Practice Stress Reduction: Engage in relaxation techniques, mindfulness, or hobbies that bring you joy and relaxation.

6. Coping with Uncertainty

MS is an unpredictable condition, and uncertainty about the future can be challenging for both the individual with MS and their caregivers. Coping with uncertainty involves:

A. Communication: Maintain open and honest communication with your loved one about their concerns and preferences for the future.

B. Planning: While it's impossible to predict every outcome, discussing future care preferences, legal matters, and end-of-life decisions can provide a sense of control.

C. Resilience: Developing resilience by focusing on the present, finding sources of strength, and seeking support can help both caregivers and their loved ones cope with uncertainty.

7. Community and Resources

Caregivers can benefit from connecting with their local MS community and accessing available resources. Support groups, both in-person and online, provide a platform for sharing experiences and seeking advice from others in similar situations. National MS organizations often offer educational materials, workshops, and assistance programs tailored to caregivers' needs.

8. Celebrating Achievements

While MS can present numerous challenges, it's essential to celebrate achievements, no matter how small they may seem. Recognize and appreciate the resilience and strength of your loved one as well as your own dedication and caregiving efforts. These celebrations can bring positivity and motivation to your journey together.

Conclusion: A Shared Journey

Caring for a loved one with MS is a shared journey that involves understanding, empathy, and self-care. Both caregivers and individuals with MS face unique challenges, but with support, open communication, and a focus on well-being, this journey can be one of love, growth, and resilience. As we conclude our exploration of MS in this book, we hope this chapter provides valuable insights and guidance for caregivers, recognizing the vital role they play in the lives of individuals with MS.

CHAPTER 10

Looking Ahead - Hope and Future Directions in Multiple Sclerosis

In this final chapter of our book on multiple sclerosis (MS), we will explore the future of MS research, treatments, and the collective hope for a world without this challenging condition. While living with MS presents significant hurdles, the ongoing advancements in research and the unwavering spirit of individuals and the MS community offer hope for a brighter future.

1. Promising Areas of Research

The landscape of MS research is continuously evolving, with several promising areas of exploration that offer hope for improved treatments and, ultimately, a cure:

A. Precision Medicine: Personalized treatments tailored to an individual's specific disease characteristics and genetic makeup are a focus of research. This approach aims to maximize treatment effectiveness while minimizing side effects.

B. Immune Modulation: A deeper understanding of the immune system's role in MS has led to the development of novel therapies that target specific immune cells and pathways involved in the disease. These treatments seek to suppress harmful immune responses while preserving the body's ability to fight infections.

C. Remyelination: Researchers are investigating strategies to promote the repair and remyelination of damaged nerves in the central nervous system. These approaches could potentially restore lost function in individuals with MS.

D. Disease Biomarkers: Biomarkers—specific biological indicators—are being studied to predict disease progression, treatment response, and relapse risk. Identifying reliable biomarkers could significantly improve treatment decisions.

E. Gut-Brain Connection: Emerging research suggests a link between the gut microbiome and MS. Investigating the role of gut bacteria in immune regulation and inflammation may open new avenues for treatment.

F.   Preventive Strategies: Studies are exploring preventive measures, such as vaccines or early interventions, to reduce the risk of developing MS in individuals at high risk.

2.   Disease-Modifying Therapies (DMTs)

The field of DMTs for MS continues to advance, offering more options and improved efficacy. DMTs are designed to modify the course of the disease and reduce the frequency and severity of relapses. Ongoing research focuses on enhancing the safety and effectiveness of these therapies, expanding treatment options, and developing strategies for progressive forms of MS.

3. Emerging Therapies and Clinical Trials

Clinical trials play a pivotal role in testing the safety and effectiveness of new treatments and therapies for MS. Participating in clinical trials provides individuals with access to cutting-edge treatments and contributes to the collective knowledge of the disease. Researchers are exploring innovative therapies, including stem cell transplantation, neuroprotective agents, and combination therapies, which hold promise for improved outcomes.

4. Advances in Imaging and Monitoring

Advances in imaging technology, such as high-resolution MRI and other neuroimaging techniques, are providing more detailed insights into the disease's progression and activity. These tools are invaluable for monitoring treatment responses and assessing disease activity, helping healthcare providers make informed decisions about MS management.

5. Telemedicine and Remote Monitoring

The COVID-19 pandemic accelerated the adoption of telemedicine in MS care. Telehealth allows individuals with MS to access healthcare remotely, reducing barriers to regular check-ups and consultations. Remote monitoring tools, including wearable devices and smartphone apps, enable individuals to track their symptoms and share data with healthcare providers for better disease management.

6. Wellness and Lifestyle Interventions

Complementary approaches to MS management are gaining recognition. Lifestyle interventions, including diet, exercise, stress reduction, and mindfulness, are being studied for their impact on symptom management and overall well-being. Integrating these strategies into MS care can enhance the quality of life.

7. Supportive Care and Mental Health

Recognizing the importance of holistic care, there is a growing emphasis on addressing the mental health and overall well-being of individuals with MS. Supportive care programs and mental health services are becoming integral components of MS management.

8. Access to Treatment and Healthcare Equity

Ensuring equitable access to MS treatments and care is a critical focus in the field. Efforts are being made to address disparities in access, especially among underserved populations, and to advocate for policies that promote affordability and accessibility of treatments.

9. Hope and Advocacy

The MS community, comprised of individuals, caregivers, healthcare providers, advocacy organizations, and researchers, remains united in its pursuit of improved treatments and, ultimately, a cure. The power of advocacy, awareness campaigns, and fundraising initiatives is driving research forward and shaping the future of MS care.

10. A Collective Vision: A World Without MS

While MS presents significant challenges, the collective vision of the MS community remains steadfast: a world without MS. Through collaboration, research, advocacy, and support, this vision continues to inspire hope and progress.

Conclusion: Embracing Hope

As we conclude our journey through this book on multiple sclerosis, we leave you with a sense of hope and optimism for the future. MS research is advancing at an unprecedented pace, and the commitment of individuals and the MS community to overcoming the challenges of this condition is unwavering.

Living with MS can be difficult, but it's important to remember that individuals with MS are resilient, and their stories are filled with courage and determination. Through understanding, support, and a shared commitment to a world without MS, we can collectively work toward improved treatments, enhanced quality of life, and, one day, a cure for this complex condition.

In the face of adversity, the MS community stands united, fueled by the hope for a brighter and healthier future for all those affected by multiple sclerosis.

CONCLUSION

A Journey Through Multiple Sclerosis

In this book, we've embarked on a comprehensive journey through the intricate landscape of multiple sclerosis (MS). Together, we've explored the science behind the disease, delved into its symptoms and diagnoses, examined the intricacies of treatment and management, and uncovered the emotional and practical aspects of living with MS. Through every chapter, we've sought to shed light on the challenges faced by individuals with MS and their loved ones, while also emphasizing the resilience and strength that characterize the MS community.

Throughout this journey, several key themes have emerged:

1. Resilience in the Face of Adversity: The individuals living with MS, their caregivers, and the entire MS community embody remarkable resilience. They face the daily challenges of this unpredictable condition with unwavering determination and courage.

2. The Power of Knowledge: Understanding MS, from its scientific underpinnings to its management strategies, is empowering. Knowledge is a critical tool for both individuals with MS and their caregivers to make informed decisions and advocate for the best possible care.

3. Support and Community: The importance of a robust support network cannot be overstated. Whether it's through healthcare providers, family, friends, or support groups, the MS community offers invaluable support, guidance, and empathy.

4. Hope and Progress: Despite the complexities of MS, hope remains a driving force. Advances in research, treatment options, and the collective vision of a world without MS inspire optimism and determination.

As we conclude this book, we want to leave you with a resounding message of hope. MS is a challenging condition, but it is one that can be faced with resilience, support, and knowledge. Whether you are an individual living with MS, a caregiver, a healthcare provider, or someone seeking to understand and support those with MS, know that you are not alone on this journey.

The future of MS care holds great promise. Research is advancing, treatments are improving, and the MS community is advocating for equity, awareness, and research funding. Together, we move forward with the collective hope of a world where MS is better understood, more effectively managed, and ultimately cured.

In closing, let this book serve as a testament to the strength of the human spirit and the power of collective efforts. With knowledge, support, and unwavering hope, we can navigate the challenges of multiple sclerosis and, together, shape a brighter future for all those touched by this condition.

www.ingramcontent.com/pod-product-compliance
Lightning Source LLC
Chambersburg PA
CBHW050728260726
48661CB00001B/117